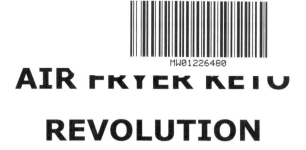

# AIR FRYER KETO
# REVOLUTION

## Delicious Meal Plans to Shed Weight, Heal Your Body, and Regain Confidence

KetonUSA

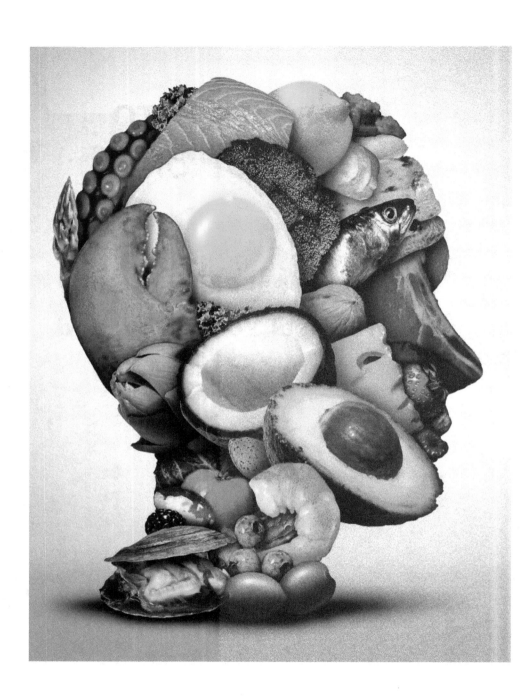

# Table of Contents

# Greek Lamb Meatballs

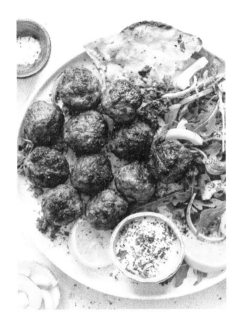

**Preparation time:** 10 minutes

**Cooking time:** 8 minutes

**Servings:** 10

### Ingredients:

- 4 ounces lamb meat, minced
- Salt and black pepper to the taste
- 1 slice of bread, toasted and crumbled 2
- tablespoons feta cheese, crumbled 1/2
- tablespoon lemon peel, grated

- 1 tablespoon oregano, chopped

## Directions:

1. In a bowl, combine meat with bread crumbs, salt, pepper, feta, oregano and lemon peel, stir well, shape 10 meatballs and place them in you air fryer.
2. Cook at 400 degrees F for 8 minutes, arrange them on a platter and serve as an appetizer. Enjoy!

**Nutrition:** calories 234, fat 12, fiber 2, carbs 20, protein 30

# Beef Party Rolls

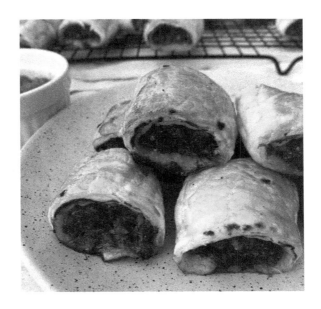

**Preparation time:** 10 minutes

**Cooking time:** 15 minutes

**Servings:** 4

**Ingredients:**

- 14 ounces beef stock
- 7 ounces white wine
- 4 beef cutlets

- Salt and black pepper to the taste 8 sage leaves
- 4 ham slices
- 1 tablespoon butter, melted

**Directions:**

1. Heat up a pan with the stock over medium high heat, add wine, cook until it reduces, take off heat and divide into small bowls
2. Season cutlets with salt and pepper, cover with sage and roll each in ham slices.
3. Brush rolls with butter, place them in your air fryer's basket and cook at 400 degrees F for 15 minutes.
4. Arrange rolls on a platter and serve them with the gravy on the side.
   Enjoy!

**Nutrition:** calories 260, fat 12, fiber 1, carbs 22, protein 21

# Pork Rolls

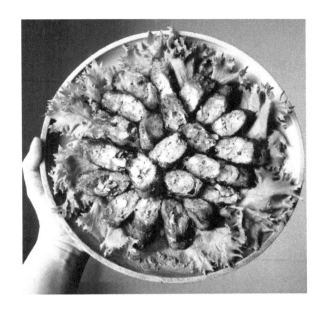

**Preparation time:** 10 minutes

**Cooking time:** 40 minutes

**Servings:** 4

**Ingredients:**

- 1 15 ounces pork fillet
- 1/2 teaspoon chili powder
- 1 teaspoon cinnamon powder
- 1 garlic clove, minced
- Salt and black pepper to the taste 2 tablespoons olive oil

- 1 and 1/2 teaspoon cumin, ground 1 red onion, chopped
- 3 tablespoons parsley, chopped

## Directions:

1. In a bowl, mix cinnamon with garlic, salt, pepper, chili powder, oil, onion, parsley and cumin and stir well
2. Put pork fillet on a cutting board, flatten it using a meat tenderizer. And use a meat tenderizer to flatten it.
3. Spread onion mix on pork, roll tight, cut into medium rolls, place them in your preheated air fryer at 360 degrees F and cook them for 35 minutes.
4. Arrange them on a platter and serve as an appetizer
   Enjoy!
   **Nutrition:** calories 304, fat 12, fiber 1, carbs 15, protein 23

# Beef Patties

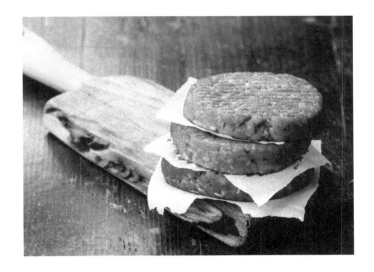

**Preparation time:** 10 minutes

**Cooking time:** 8 minutes

**Servings:** 4

**Ingredients:**

- 14 ounces beef, minced
- 2 tablespoons ham, cut into strips 1 leek, chopped
- 3 tablespoons bread crumbs
- Salt and black pepper to the taste 1/2 teaspoon nutmeg, ground

---

## Directions:

1. In a bowl, mix beef with leek, salt, pepper, ham, breadcrumbs and nutmeg, stir well and shape small patties out of this mix.
2. Place them in your air fryer's basket, cook at 400 degrees F for 8 minutes, arrange on a platter and serve as an appetizer.
   Enjoy!

**Nutrition:** calories 260, fat 12, fiber 3, carbs 12, protein 21

# Roasted Bell Pepper Rolls

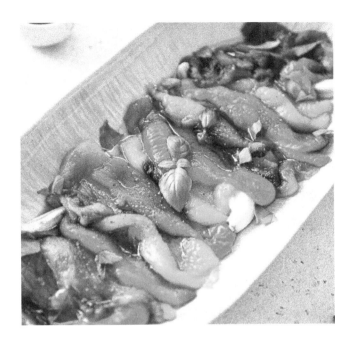

**Preparation time:** 10 minutes

**Cooking time:** 10 minutes

**Servings:** 8

**Ingredients:**

- 1 yellow bell pepper, halved
- 1 orange bell pepper, halved

- Salt and black pepper to the taste 4 ounces feta cheese, crumbled 1 green onion, chopped 2 tablespoons oregano, chopped

**Directions:**

1. In a bowl, mix cheese with onion, oregano, salt and pepper and whisk well.
2. Place bell pepper halves in your air fryer's basket, cook at 400 degrees F for 10 minutes, transfer to a cutting board, cool down and peel.
3. Divide cheese mix on each bell pepper half, roll, secure with toothpicks, arrange on a platter and serve as an appetizer.
   Enjoy!
   **Nutrition:** calories 170, fat 1, fiber 2, carbs 8, protein 5

# Stuffed Peppers

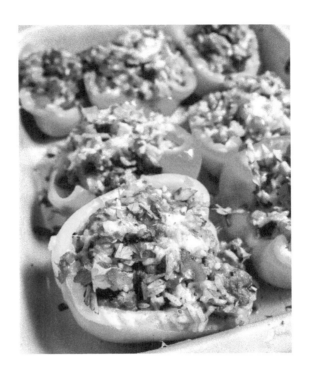

**Preparation time:** 10 minutes

**Cooking time:** 8 minutes

**Servings:** 8

**Ingredients:**

- 8 small bell peppers, tops cut off and seeds removed 1 tablespoon olive oil
- Salt and black pepper to the taste

- 3.5 ounces goat cheese, cut into 8 pieces

**Directions:**

1. In a bowl, mix cheese with oil with salt and pepper and toss to coat.
2. Stuff each pepper with goat cheese, place them in your air fryer's basket, cook at 400 degrees F for 8 minutes.
3. Arrange on a platter and serve as an appetizer.

   Enjoy!

   **Nutrition:** calories 120, fat 1, fiber 1, carbs 12, protein 8

# Herbed Tomatoes Appetizer

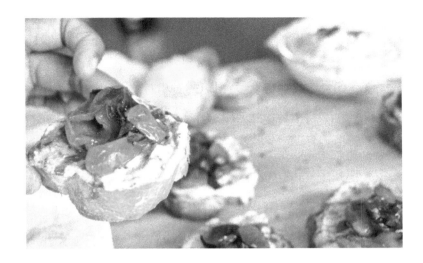

**Preparation time:** 10 minutes

**Cooking time:** 20 minutes

**Servings:** 2

**Ingredients:**

- 2 tomatoes, halved
- Cooking spray
- Salt and black pepper to the taste 1 teaspoon parsley, dried
- 1 teaspoon basil, dried
- 1 teaspoon oregano, dried

- 1 teaspoon rosemary, dried

## Directions:

1. Spray tomato halves with cooking oil, season with salt, pepper, parsley, basil, oregano and rosemary over them.
2. Place them in your air fryer's basket and cook at 320 degrees F for 20 minutes. Arrange them on a platter and serve as an appetizer. Enjoy!

**Nutrition:** calories 100, fat 1, fiber 1, carbs 4, protein 1

# Olives Balls

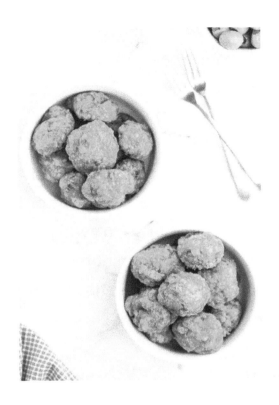

**Preparation time:** 10 minutes

**Cooking time:** 4 minutes

**Servings:** 6

**Ingredients:**

- 8 black olives, pitted and minced Salt and black pepper to the taste

- 2 tablespoons sun dried tomato pesto
- 14 pepperoni slices, chopped
- 4 ounces cream cheese
- 1 tablespoons basil, chopped

**Directions:**

1. In a bowl, mix cream cheese with salt, pepper, basil, pepperoni, pesto and black olives, stir well and shape small balls out of this mix.
2. Place them in your air fryer's basket, cook at 350 degrees F for 4 minutes, arrange on a platter and serve as a snack.
   Enjoy!

**Nutrition:** calories 100, fat 1, fiber 0, carbs 8, protein 3

# Jalapeno Balls

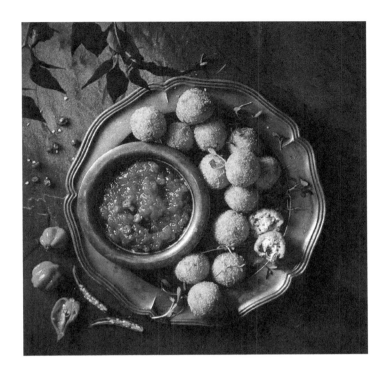

**Preparation time:** 10 minutes

**Cooking time:** 4 minutes

**Servings:** 3

**Ingredients:**

- 3 bacon slices, cooked and crumbled 3 ounces cream cheese
- 1/4 teaspoon onion powder

- Salt and black pepper to the taste
- 1 jalapeno pepper, chopped 1/2 teaspoon parsley, dried 1/4 teaspoon garlic powder

**Directions:**

1. In a bowl, mix cream cheese with jalapeno pepper, onion and garlic powder, parsley, bacon salt and pepper and stir well.
2. Shape small balls out of this mix, place them in your air fryer's basket.
3. Cook at 350 degrees F for 4 minutes, arrange on a platter and serve as an appetizer.

Enjoy!

**Nutrition:** calories 172, fat 4, fiber 1, carbs 12, protein 5

# Wrapped Shrimp

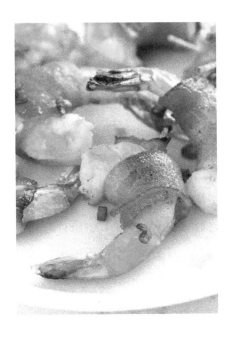

**Preparation time:** 10 minutes

**Cooking time:** 8 minutes

**Servings:** 16

**Ingredients:**

- 2 tablespoons olive oil
- 10 ounces already cooked shrimp, peeled and deveined 1 tablespoons mint, chopped
- 1/3 cup blackberries, ground

- 11 prosciutto sliced
- 1/3 cup red wine

## Directions:

1. Wrap each shrimp in a prosciutto slices, drizzle the oil over them, rub well.
2. Place in your preheated air fryer at 390 degrees F and fry them for 8 minutes.
3. Meanwhile, heat up a pan with ground blackberries over medium heat, add mint and wine, stir, cook for 3 minutes and take off heat.
4. Arrange shrimp on a platter, drizzle blackberries sauce over them and serve as an appetizer.
   Enjoy!

**Nutrition:** calories 224, fat 12, fiber 2, carbs 12, protein 14

# Broccoli Patties

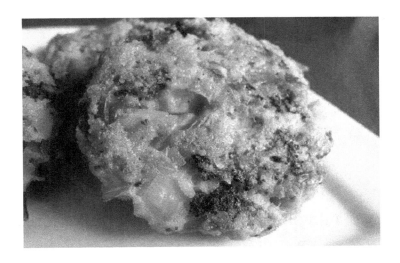

**Preparation time:** 10 minutes

**Cooking time:** 10 minutes

**Servings:** 12

### Ingredients:

- 4 cups broccoli florets
- 1 and 1/2 cup almond flour
- 1 teaspoon paprika
- Salt and black pepper to the taste 2 eggs
- 1/4 cup olive oil

- 2 cups cheddar cheese, grated1 teaspoon garlic powder
- 1/2 teaspoon apple cider vinegar 1/2 teaspoon baking soda

## Directions:

1. Put broccoli florets in your food processor, add salt and pepper, blend well and transfer to a bowl.
2. Add almond flour, salt, pepper, paprika, garlic powder, baking soda, cheese, oil, eggs and vinegar, stir well and shape 12 patties out of this mix.
3. Place them in your preheated air fryer's basket and cook at 350 degrees F for 10 minutes.
4. Arrange patties on a platter and serve as an appetizer.
   Enjoy!

**Nutrition:** calories 203, fat 12, fiber 2, carbs 14, protein 2

# Different Stuffed Peppers

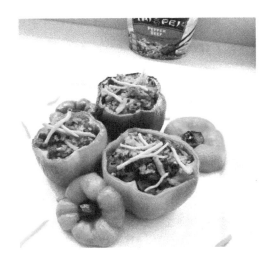

**Preparation time:** 10 minutes

**Cooking time:** 20 minutes

**Servings:** 6

**Ingredients:**

- 1 pound mini bell peppers, halved Salt and black pepper to the taste 1 teaspoon garlic powder
- 1 teaspoon sweet paprika
- 1/2 teaspoon oregano, dried
  1/4 teaspoon red pepper flakes

1 pound beef meat, ground

1 and 1/2 cups cheddar cheese, shredded 1 tablespoons chili powder

1 teaspoon cumin, ground

Sour cream for serving

## Directions:

1. In a bowl, mix chili powder with paprika, salt, pepper, cumin, oregano, pepper flakes and garlic powder and stir.
2. Heat up a pan over medium heat, add beef, stir and brown for 10 minutes.
3. Add chili powder mix, stir, take off heat and stuff pepper halves with this mix.
4. Sprinkle cheese all over, place peppers in your air fryer's basket and cook them at 350 degrees F for 6 minutes.
5. Arrange peppers on a platter and serve them with sour cream on the side.

Enjoy!

**Nutrition:** calories 170, fat 22, fiber 3, carbs 6, protein 27

# Cheesy Zucchini Snack

**Preparation time:** 10 minutes

**Cooking time:** 8 minutes

**Servings:** 4 **Ingredients:**

- 1 cup mozzarella, shredded
- 1/4 cup tomato sauce
- 1 zucchini, sliced
- Salt and black pepper to the taste A pinch of cumin Cooking spray

**Directions:**

1. Arrange zucchini slices in your air fryer's basket.
2. Spray them with cooking oil, spread tomato sauce all over, them, season with salt, pepper, cumin, sprinkle mozzarella at the end. Cook them at 320 degrees F for 8 minutes.
3. Arrange them on a platter and serve as a snack. Enjoy!
   **Nutrition:** calories 150, fat 4, fiber 2, carbs 12, protein 4

# Spinach Balls

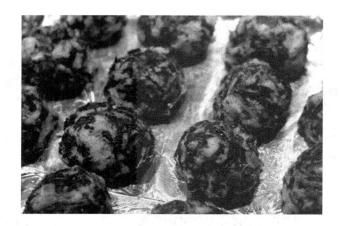

**Preparation time:** 10 minutes

**Cooking time:** 7 minutes

**Servings:** 30

**Ingredients:**

- 4 tablespoons butter, melted 2 eggs
- 1 cup flour
- 16 ounces spinach
- 1/3 cup feta cheese, crumbled
- 1/4 teaspoon nutmeg, ground
- 1/3 cup parmesan, grated
- Salt and black pepper to the taste

- 1 tablespoon onion powder
- 3 tablespoons whipping cream
- 1 teaspoon garlic powder

## Directions:

1. In your blender, mix spinach with butter, eggs, flour, feta cheese, parmesan, nutmeg, whipping cream, salt, pepper, onion and garlic pepper, blend very well and keep in the freezer for 10 minutes.
2. Shape 30 spinach balls, place them in your air fryer's basket and cook at 300 degrees F for 7 minutes.
3. Serve as a party appetizer. Enjoy!

**Nutrition:** calories 60, fat 5, fiber 1, carbs 1, protein 2

# Mushrooms Appetizer

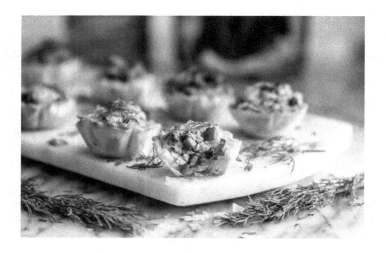

**Preparation time:** 10 minutes

**Cooking time:** 10 minutes

**Servings:** 4

**Ingredients:**

- 1/4 cup mayonnaise
- 1 teaspoon garlic powder
- 1 small yellow onion, chopped
- 24 ounces white mushroom caps
- Salt and black pepper to the taste
- 1 teaspoon curry powder

- 4 ounces cream cheese, soft
- 1/4 cup sour cream
- 1/2 cup Mexican cheese, shredded
- 1 cup shrimp, cooked, peeled, deveined and chopped

**Directions:**

1. In a bowl, mix mayo with garlic powder, onion, curry powder, cream cheese, sour cream, Mexican cheese, shrimp, salt and pepper to the taste and whisk well.
2. Stuff mushrooms with this mix, place them in your air fryer's basket and cook at 300 degrees F for 10 minutes.
3. Arrange on a platter and serve as an appetizer.
   Enjoy!

   **Nutrition:** calories 200, fat 20, fiber 3, carbs 16, protein 14

# Cheesy Party Wings

**Preparation time:** 10 minutes

**Cooking time:** 12 minutes

**Servings:** 6

**Ingredients:**

- 6 pound chicken wings, halved Salt and black pepper to the taste 1/2 teaspoon Italian seasoning
- 2 tablespoons butter
- 1/2 cup parmesan cheese, grated
- A pinch of red pepper flakes, crushed 1 teaspoon garlic powder
- 1 egg

**Directions:**

1. Arrange chicken wings in your air fryer's basket and cook at 390 degrees F and cook for 9 minutes.
2. Meanwhile, in your blender, mix butter with cheese, egg, salt, pepper, pepper flakes, garlic

powder and Italian seasoning and blend very well.

3. Take chicken wings out, pour cheese sauce over them, toss to coat well and cook in your air fryer's basket at 390 degrees F for 3 minutes.
4. Serve them as an appetizer.
   Enjoy!

**Nutrition:** calories 204, fat 8, fiber 1, carbs 18, protein 14

# Cheese Sticks

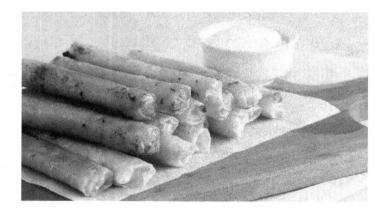

**Preparation time:** 1 hour and 10 minutes

**Cooking time:** 8 minutes

**Servings:** 16

**Ingredients:**

- 2 eggs, whisked
- Salt and black pepper to the taste
- 8 mozzarella cheese strings, cut into halves 1 cup parmesan, grated
- 1 tablespoon Italian seasoning
- Cooking spray
- 1 garlic clove, minced

## Directions:

1. In a bowl, mix parmesan with salt, pepper, Italian seasoning and garlic and stir well.
2. Put whisked eggs in another bowl.
3. Dip mozzarella sticks in egg mixture, then in cheese mix.
4. Dip them again in egg and in parmesan mix and keep them in the freezer for 1 hour.
5. Spray cheese sticks with cooking oil, place them in your air fryer's basket and cook at 390 degrees F for 8 minutes flipping them halfway.
6. Arrange them on a platter and serve as an appetizer.
   Enjoy!

**Nutrition:** calories 140, fat 5, fiber 1, carbs 3, protein 4

# Sweet Bacon Snack

**Preparation time:** 10 minutes

**Cooking time:** 30 minutes

**Servings:** 16

**Ingredients:**

- 1/2 teaspoon cinnamon powder 16 bacon slices
- 1 tablespoon avocado oil
- 3 ounces dark chocolate
- 1 teaspoon maple extract

**Directions:**

1. Arrange bacon slices in your air fryer's basket, sprinkle cinnamon mix over them and cook them at 300 degrees F for 30 minutes.
2. Heat up a pot with the oil over medium heat, add chocolate and stir until it melts. Add maple extract, stir, take off heat and leave aside to cool down a bit.
3. Take bacon strips out of the oven, leave them to cool down, dip each in chocolate mix, place

them on a parchment paper and leave them to cool down completely.

4. Serve cold as a snack.

Enjoy!

**Nutrition:** calories 200, fat 4, fiber 5, carbs 12, protein 3

# Chicken Rolls

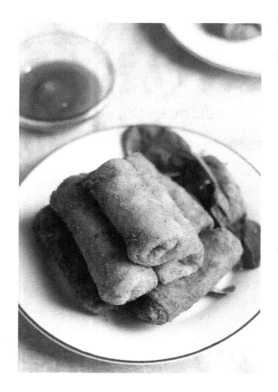

**Preparation time:** 2 hours and 10 minutes

**Cooking time:** 10 minutes

**Servings:** 12

**Ingredients:**

- 4 ounces blue cheese, crumbled

- 2 cups chicken, cooked and chopped Salt and black pepper to the taste
- 2 green onions, chopped
- 2 celery stalks, finely chopped
- 1/2 cup tomato sauce
- 12 egg roll wrappers
- Cooking spray

**Directions:**

1. In a bowl, mix chicken meat with blue cheese, salt, pepper, green onions, celery and tomato sauce, stir well and keep in the fridge for 2 hours.
2. Place egg wrappers on a working surface, divide chicken mix on them, roll and seal edges.
3. Place rolls in your air fryer's basket, spray them with cooking oil and cook at 350 degrees F for 10 minutes, flipping them halfway. Enjoy!

**Nutrition:** calories 220, fat 7, fiber 2, carbs 14, protein 10

# Tasty Kale and Celery Crackers

**Preparation time:** 10 minutes

**Cooking time:** 20 minutes

**Servings:** 6

**Ingredients:**

- 2 cups flax seed, ground
- 2 cups flax seed, soaked overnight and
- drained 4 bunches kale, chopped
- 1 bunch basil, chopped
- 1/2 bunch celery, chopped
- 4 garlic cloves, minced
- 1/3 cup olive oil

**Directions:**

1. In your food processor mix ground flaxseed with celery, kale, basil and garlic and blend well.
2. Add oil and soaked flaxseed and blend again, spread in your air fryer's pan, cut into medium crackers and cook them at 380 degrees F for 20 minutes.

---

3. Divide into bowls and serve as an appetizer.
   Enjoy!

   **Nutrition:** calories 143, fat 1, fiber 2, carbs 8,
   protein 4

# Egg White Chips

**Preparation time:** 5 minutes

**Cooking time:** 8 minutes

**Servings:** 2

**Ingredients:**

- 1/2 tablespoon water
- 2 tablespoons parmesan, shredded 4 eggs whites
- Salt and black pepper to the taste

**Directions:**

1. In a bowl, mix egg whites with salt, pepper and water and whisk well.
2. Spoon this into a muffin pan that fits your air fryer, sprinkle cheese on top, introduce in your air fryer and cook at 350 degrees F for 8 minutes.
3. Arrange egg white chips on a platter and serve as a snack. Enjoy!
   **Nutrition:** calories 180, fat 2, fiber 1, carbs 12, protein 7

# Tuna Cakes

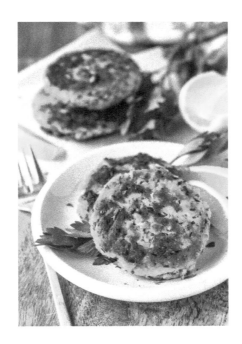

**Preparation time:** 10 minutes

**Cooking time:** 10 minutes

**Servings:** 12

**Ingredients:**

- 15 ounces canned tuna, drain and flaked 3 eggs
- 1/2 teaspoon dill, dried
- 1 teaspoon parsley, dried

- 1/2 cup red onion, chopped
- 1 teaspoon garlic powder
- Salt and black pepper to the taste Cooking spray

## Directions:

1. In a bowl, mix tuna with salt, pepper, dill, parsley, onion, garlic powder and eggs, stir well and shape medium cakes out of this mix.
2. Place tuna cakes in your air fryer's basket, spray them with cooking oil and cook at 350 degrees F for 10 minutes, flipping them halfway.
3. Arrange them on a platter and serve as an appetizer.
   Enjoy!

**Nutrition:** calories 140, fat 2, fiber 1, carbs 8, protein 6

# Calamari and Shrimp Snack

**Preparation time:** 10 minutes

**Cooking time:** 20 minutes

**Servings:** 1

**Ingredients:**

- 8 ounces calamari, cut into medium rings 7 ounces shrimp, peeled and deveined
- 1 egg
- 3 tablespoons white flour
- 1 tablespoon olive oil
- 2 tablespoons avocado, chopped 1 teaspoon tomato paste
- 1 tablespoon mayonnaise
- A splash of Worcestershire sauce 1 teaspoon lemon juice
- Salt and black pepper to the taste
- 1/2teaspoon turmeric powder

## Directions:

1. In a bowl, whisk egg with oil, add calamari rings and shrimp and toss to coat. In another bowl, mix flour with salt, pepper and turmeric and stir.

2. Dredge calamari and shrimp in this mix, place them in your air fryer's basket and cook at 350 degrees F for 9 minutes, flipping them once.

3. Meanwhile, in a bowl, mix avocado with mayo and tomato paste and mash using a fork.

4. Add Worcestershire sauce, lemon juice, salt and pepper and stir well.

5. Arrange calamari and shrimp on a platter and serve with the sauce on the side.
   Enjoy!

**Nutrition:** calories 288, fat 23, fiber 3, carbs 10, protein 15

# Loaded Roasted Broccoli

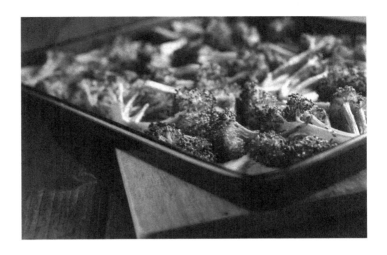

If you've ever thought broccoli was boring, this recipe will change your mind forever. It's stuffed to the gills with savory flavor and delicious fats to help keep you full, not to mention the great protein boost that comes from the broccoli itself!

- **Hands On Time**: 10 minutes

- **Cook Time**: 10 minutes

**Serves** 2

## Ingredients:

- 3 cups fresh broccoli florets

- 1 tablespoon coconut oil

- 1/2 cup shredded sharp Cheddar cheese

- 1/4 cup full-fat sour cream 4 slices sugar-free bacon, cooked and crumbled 1 scallion, sliced on the bias

### Directions

1. Place broccoli into the air fryer basket and drizzle it with coconut oil.
   Adjust the temperature to 350°F and set the timer for 10 minutes.
2. Toss the basket two or three times during cooking to avoid burned spots.
3. When broccoli begins to crisp at ends, remove from fryer.
4. Top with shredded cheese, sour cream, and crumbled bacon and garnish with scallion slices.

## PER SERVING

Calories: 361 Protein: 18.4 G
Fiber: 3.6 G
Net Carbohydrates: 6.9 G Fat: 25.7 G Sodium: 564
Mg Carbohydrates: 10.5 G Sugar: 3.3 G

# Garlic Herb Butter Roasted Radishes

When roasted, radishes make a surprisingly excellent red potato substitute. When roasted in an air fryer, the crisp you're able to achieve is incomparable. Full of health benefits like vitamin C and healthy fiber, this is one side dish you'll always feel good about eating!

- **Hands On Time**: 10 minutes

- **Cook Time**: 10 minutes

**Serves** 4

**Ingredients:**

- 1 pound radishes

- 2 tablespoons unsalted butter, melted

- 1/2 teaspoon garlic powder

- 1/2 teaspoon dried parsley

- 1/4 teaspoon dried oregano

- 1/4 teaspoon ground black pepper

## Directions

1. Remove roots from radishes and cut into quarters.
2. In a small bowl, add butter and seasonings. Toss the radishes in the herb butter and place into the air fryer basket.
3. Adjust the temperature to 350°F and set the timer for 10 minutes.
4. Halfway through the cooking time, toss the radishes in the air fryer basket. Continue cooking until edges begin to turn brown. Serve warm.

## PER SERVING

Calories: 63
Protein: 0.7 G Fiber: 1.3 G
Net Carbohydrates: 1.6 G Fat: 5.4 G
Sodium: 28 Mg Carbohydrates: 2.9 G Sugar: 1.4 G

# Sausage-Stuffed Mushroom Caps

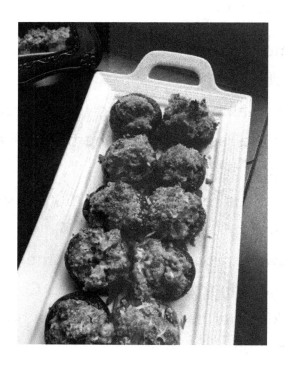

Mushrooms are very low-carb, are high in potassium, and have a fresh, earthy taste. Stuffing them with sausage boosts their protein and fat contents, and more importantly it elevates their flavor to something you won't be able to get enough of!

- **Hands On Time**: 10 minutes

- **Cook Time**: 8 minutes

**Serves** 2

**Ingredients:**

- 6 large portobello mushroom caps

- 1/2 pound Italian sausage

- 1/4 cup chopped onion

- 2 tablespoons blanched finely ground almond flour

- 1/4 cup grated Parmesan cheese

- 1 teaspoon minced fresh garlic

## Directions

1. Use a spoon to hollow out each mushroom cap, reserving scrapings.
2. In a medium skillet over medium heat, brown the sausage about 10 minutes or until fully cooked and no pink remains.
3. Drain and then add reserved mushroom scrapings, onion, almond flour, Parmesan, and garlic.

4.  Gently fold ingredients together and continue cooking an additional minute, then remove from heat.

5.  Evenly spoon the mixture into mushroom caps and place the caps into a 6" round pan.

6.  Place pan into the air fryer basket.

7.  Adjust the temperature to 375°F and set the timer for 8 minutes.

8.  When finished cooking, the tops will be browned and bubbling. Serve warm.

## PER SERVING

Calories: 404
Protein: 24.3 G Fiber: 4.5 G
Net Carbohydrates: 13.7 G Fat: 25.8 G
Sodium: 1,106 Mg Carbohydrates: 18.2 G Sugar: 8.1 G

# Cheesy Cauliflower Tots

With the carb count in potatoes being so high, tater tots would be very difficult to fit into your macros. Luckily, cauliflower is a great substitute to give you that same crispy texture for a wonderfully kid-friendly side dish. Serve these warm with low- carb ketchup or your favorite dipping sauce.

- **Hands On Time**: 15 minutes

- **Cook Time**: 12 minutes

**Yields** 16 tots (4 per serving)

**Ingredients:**

- 1 large head cauliflower

- 1 cup shredded mozzarella cheese

- 1/2 cup grated Parmesan cheese 1 large egg

- 1/4 teaspoon garlic powder

- 1/4 teaspoon dried parsley

- 1/8 teaspoon onion powder

## Directions

1. On the stovetop, fill a large pot with 2 cups water and place a steamer in the pan. Bring water to a boil. Cut the cauliflower into florets and place on steamer basket. Cover pot with lid.

2. Allow cauliflower to steam 7 minutes until fork tender.

3. Remove from steamer basket and place into cheesecloth or clean kitchen towel and let cool.

4. Squeeze over sink to remove as much excess moisture as possible.

5. The mixture will be too soft to form into tots if not all the moisture is removed. Mash with a fork to a smooth consistency.

6. Put the cauliflower into a large mixing bowl and add mozzarella, Parmesan, egg, garlic powder, parsley, and onion powder. Stir until fully combined. The mixture should be wet but easy to mold.

7. Take 2 tablespoons of the mixture and roll into tot shape. Repeat with remaining mixture. Place into the air fryer basket.

8. Adjust the temperature to 320°F and set the timer for 12 minutes.

9. Turn tots halfway through the cooking time. Cauliflower tots should be golden when fully cooked. Serve warm.

## PER SERVING

Calories: 181 Protein: 13.5 G Fiber: 3.0 G
Net Carbohydrates: 6.6 G Fat: 9.5 G Sodium: 417
Mg Carbohydrates: 9.6 G Sugar: 3.2 G

# Kid Friendly!

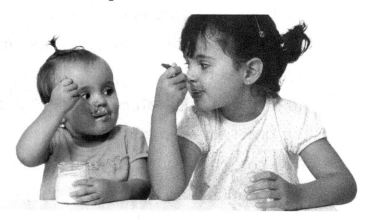

These are great to make for kids because they look just like a classic tater tot, but they're much better for you. The cheese also helps to mask the cauliflower taste, making this the ultimate way to sneak veggies in! Remove all loose leaves from Brussels sprouts and cut each in half.

Drizzle sprouts with coconut oil and place into the air fryer basket. Adjust the temperature to 400°F and set the timer for 10 minutes. You may want to gently stir halfway through the cooking time, depending on how they are beginning to brown. When completely cooked, they should be tender with darker caramelized spots. Remove from fryer basket and drizzle with melted butter. Serve immediately.

# Crispy Brussels Sprouts

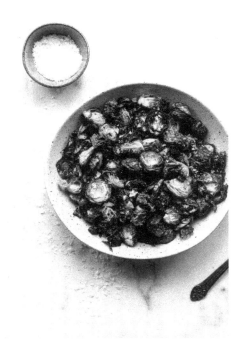

Get ready to cook some Brussels sprouts your kids will be excited about eating! They're rich in nutrients, including heart- healthy omega-3 fatty acids. This version is a complete reversal of the bland and boring Brussels sprouts you grew up eating!

- **Hands On Time**: 5 minutes

- **Cook Time**: 10 minutes

**Serves** 4

- 1 pound Brussels sprouts

- 1 tablespoon coconut oil

- 1 tablespoon unsalted butter, melted

## Directions

## PER SERVING

Calories: 90 Protein: 2.9 G Fiber: 3.2 G Net Carbohydrates: 4.3 G Fat: 6.1 G Sodium: 21 Mg Carbohydrates: 7.5 G Sugar: 1.9 G

# Zucchini Parmesan Chips

It can be difficult to get that satisfying crunch that a lot of carb- filled foods carry, but it's easier than ever with your air fryer. These thinly sliced zucchini chips are a nutrient-rich treat for mealtime or snack time!

- **Hands On Time**: 10 minutes

- **Cook Time**: 10 minutes

**Serves** 4

**Ingredients:**

- 2 medium zucchini

- 1 ounce pork rinds

- 1/2 cup grated Parmesan cheese

- 1 large egg

### Directions

1. Slice zucchini in 1/4"-thick slices. Place between two layers of paper towels or a clean kitchen nj towel for 30 minutes to remove excess moisture.

―

2. Place pork rinds into food processor and pulse until finely ground. Pour into medium bowl and mix with Parmesan.

3. Beat egg in a small bowl.

4. Dip zucchini slices in egg and then in pork rind mixture, coating as completely as possible. Carefully place each slice into the air fryer basket in a single layer, working in batches as necessary.

5. Adjust temperature to 320°F and set the timer for 10 minutes. Flip chips halfway through the cooking time. Serve warm.

## PER SERVING

Calories: 121

Protein: 9.9 G Fiber: 0.6 G Net Carbohydrates: 3.2 G Fat: 6.7 G Sodium: 364 Mg Carbohydrates: 3.8 G Sugar: 1.6 G

# Roasted Garlic

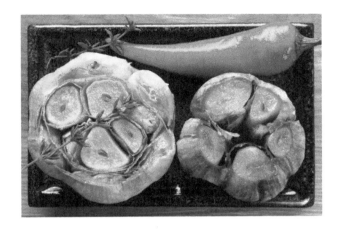

Roasted garlic is one of the easiest ways to add a boost of flavor to any dish, from chicken to mashed cauliflower to the Roasted Garlic White Zucchini Rolls in Chapter 8. Unlike traditional oven recipes, which can take over an hour to get the roasted garlic right, your air fryer can extract all the savory flavor in just minutes!

- **Hands On Time**: 5 minutes

- **Cook Time**: 20 minutes

**Yields** 12 cloves (1 per serving)

**Ingredients:**

- 1 medium head garlic

- 2 teaspoons avocado oil

**Directions**

1. Remove any hanging excess peel from the garlic but leave the cloves covered. Cut off V4 of the head of garlic, exposing the tips of the cloves.

2. Drizzle with avocado oil. Place the garlic head into a small sheet of aluminum foil, completely enclosing it. Place it into the air fryer basket.

3. Adjust the temperature to 400°F and set the timer for 20 minutes. If your garlic head is a bit smaller, check it after 15 minutes.

4. When done, garlic should be golden brown and very soft.

5. To serve, cloves should pop out and easily be spread or sliced. Store in an airtight container in the refrigerator up to 5 days.

6. You may also freeze individual cloves on a baking sheet, then store together in a freezer-safe storage bag once frozen

## PER SERVING

Calories: 11
Protein: 0.2 G
Fiber: 0.1 G
Net Carbohydrates: 0.9 G Fat: 0.7 G Sodium: 0 Mg
Carbohydrates: 1.0 G Sugar: 0.0 G

## HOW TO USE ROASTED GARLIC

Roasted garlic has a milder, sweeter taste than raw garlic, which complements many dishes. Make a quick roasted garlic and herb butter for your steak or pork chops. Simply mash a clove of roasted garlic with 1/4 cup softened butter and add your favorite herbs.

# Kale Chips

With just the right seasoning and only a few minutes in your air fryer, you'll have a crispy snack that's easy to take on the go! Plus, kale is high in fiber, helping to promote a regular and healthy digestive tract.

- **Hands On Time**: 5 minutes

- **Cook Time**: 5 minutes

**Serves** 4

**Ingredients:**

- 4 cups stemmed kale

- 2 teaspoons avocado oil

- 2 teaspoon salt

   **Directions**

   1. In a large bowl, toss kale in avocado oil and sprinkle with salt. Place into the air fryer basket.
   2. Adjust the temperature to 400°F and set the timer for 5 minutes.

---

3. Kale will be crispy when done. Serve
   immediately.

## PER SERVING

Calories: 25
Protein: 0.5 G Fiber: 0.4 G
Net Carbohydrates: 0.7 G Fat: 2.2 G
Sodium: 295 Mg Carbohydrates: 1.1 G Sugar:
0.3 G

# Buffalo Cauliflower

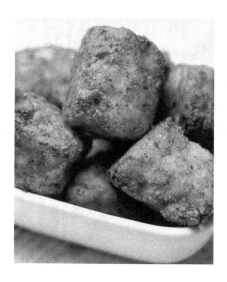

Cauliflower steaks are a great vegetarian option that have nutrients and flavor. Roasting them with buffalo sauce gives you a light and spicy dish that is totally guilt-free! Serve with crumbled blue cheese or ranch dressing if you need to tone down the spice!

- **Hands On Time**: 5 minutes

- **Cook Time**: 5 minutes

**Serves** 4

## Ingredients:

- 4 cups cauliflower florets

- 2 tablespoons salted butter, melted

- 2 (1-ounce) dry ranch seasoning packet

- 1/4 cup buffalo sauce

### Directions

1. In a large bowl, toss cauliflower with butter and dry ranch.
2. Place into the air fryer basket.
3. Adjust the temperature to 400°F and set the timer for 5 minutes.
4. Shake the basket two or three times during cooking. When tender, remove cauliflower from fryer basket and toss in buffalo sauce. Serve warm.

### PER SERVING

Calories: 87
Protein: 2.1 G Fiber: 2.1 G
Net Carbohydrates: 5.2 G Fat: 5.6 G
Sodium: 803 Mg Carbohydrates: 7.3 G Sugar: 2.1 G

# Green Bean Casserole

- **Hands On Time**: 10 minutes

- Cook Time: 15 minutes

**Serves** 4

**Ingredients:**

- 4 tablespoons unsalted butter

- 1/4 cup diced yellow onion

- 1/2 cup chopped white mushrooms

- 1/2 cup heavy whipping cream

- 1 ounce full-fat cream cheese

- 1/2 cup chicken broth

- 1/4 teaspoon xanthan gum

- 1 pound fresh green beans, edges trimmed

- 1/2 ounce pork rinds, finely ground

## Directions

1. In a medium skillet over medium heat, melt the butter. Saute the onion and mushrooms until they become soft and fragrant, about 3-5 minutes.

2. Add the heavy whipping cream, cream cheese, and broth to the pan. Whisk until smooth. Bring to a boil and then reduce to a simmer. Sprinkle the xanthan gum into the pan and remove from heat.

3. Chop the green beans into 2" pieces and place into a 4-cup round baking dish. Pour the sauce mixture over them and stir until coated. Top the dish with ground pork rinds. Place into the air fryer basket.

4. Adjust the temperature to 320°F and set the timer for 15 minutes.

5. Top will be golden and green beans fork tender when fully cooked. Serve warm.

This low-carb spin on a potluck favorite will be the newest addition to your holiday menu. You'll notice the dish is missing the cream of mushroom soup you might be used to, but don't worry; you'll get all the traditional flavor without all the unnecessary carbs!

## PER SERVING

Calories: 267 Protein: 3.6 G Fiber: 3.2 G
Net Carbohydrates: 6.5 G Fat: 23.4 G Sodium: 161
Mg Carbohydrates: 9.7 G Sugar: 5.1 G

## ARE GREEN BEANS KETO-FRIENDLY?

Green beans are legumes, but that doesn't mean you can't enjoy them on a ketogenic diet. Traditionally keto excluded legumes, including peanuts. Nowadays, a more rounded approach is taken and as long as the carbs are low and fit your macros, generally you can enjoy them. There are 3.6 grams net carbs in a 1-cup serving of green beans, which makes them a great choice!

# Cilantro Lime Roasted Cauliflower

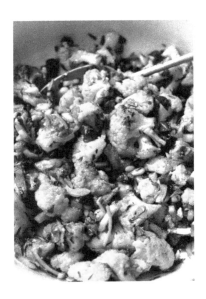

Although it's rich in nutrients, like vitamin C, cauliflower is usually a pretty bland-tasting vegetable. This gives you an excellent opportunity to flavor it just the way you like for an appetizing side. This cilantro lime flavoring will complement any steak dish perfectly!

- **Hands On Time**: 10 minutes

- **Cook Time**: 7 minutes

**Serves** 4

## Ingredients:

- 2 cups chopped cauliflower florets
- 2 tablespoons coconut oil, melted
- 2 teaspoons chili powder
- 1/2 teaspoon garlic powder
- 1 medium lime
- 2 tablespoons chopped cilantro

## Directions

1. In a large bowl, toss cauliflower with coconut oil. Sprinkle with chili powder and garlic powder. Place seasoned cauliflower into the air fryer basket.
2. Adjust the temperature to 350°F and set the timer for 7 minutes.
3. Cauliflower will be tender and begin to turn golden at the edges.
4. Place into serving bowl.
5. Cut the lime into quarters and squeeze juice over cauliflower. Garnish with cilantro.

## PER SERVING

Calories: 73
Protein: 1.1 G Fiber: 1.1 G
Net Carbohydrates: 2.2 G Fat: 6.5 G
Sodium: 16 Mg Carbohydrates: 3.3 G Sugar: 1.1 G

# Dinner Rolls

Do you miss bread on your keto diet? This low-carb substitute will satisfy any bread craving you may have and give you a great side dish to eat with your dinner. The dough can also be baked in a loaf pan or flattened out on a pizza pan to take care of you no matter which bread craving strikes!

- **Hands On Time**: 10 minutes

- **Cook Time**: 12 minutes

**Serves** 6

**Ingredients:**

- 1 cup shredded mozzarella cheese

- 1 ounce full-fat cream cheese

- 1 cup blanched finely ground almond flour

- 1/4 cup ground flaxseed

- 1/2 teaspoon baking powder

- 1 large egg

## Directions

1. Place mozzarella, cream cheese, and almond flour in a large microwave-safe bowl. Microwave for 1 minute. Mix until smooth.
2. Add flaxseed, baking powder, and egg until fully combined and smooth. Microwave an additional 15 seconds if it becomes too firm.
3. Separate the dough into six pieces and roll into balls. Place the balls into the air fryer basket.
4. Adjust the temperature to 320°F and set the timer for 12 minutes. Allow rolls to cool completely before serving.

## PER SERVING

Calories: 228 Protein: 10.8 G Fiber: 3.9 G
Net Carbohydrates: 2.9 G Fat: 18.1 G Sodium: 188
Mg Carbohydrates: 6.8 G Sugar: 1.2 G

# Coconut Flour Cheesy Garlic Biscuits

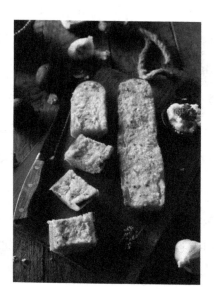

Missing biscuits on a keto diet is completely understandable. There's practically no dish they don't side perfectly with. Try these fluffy and flavorful treats with shrimp scampi for a keto-friendly at- home restaurant experience!

- **Hands On Time**: 10 minutes

- **Cook Time**: 12 minutes

**Serves** 4

## Ingredients:

- 1/3 cup coconut flour

- 1/2 teaspoon baking powder

- 1/2 teaspoon garlic powder , 1 large egg

- 1/4 cup unsalted butter, melted and divided

- 1/2 cup shredded sharp Cheddar cheese

- 1 scallion, sliced

## Directions

1. In a large bowl, mix coconut flour, baking powder, and garlic powder.

2. Stir in egg, half of the melted butter, Cheddar cheese, and scallions. Pour the mixture into a 6" round baking pan. Place into the air fryer basket. Adjust the temperature to 320°F and set the timer for 12 minutes.

3. To serve, remove from pan and allow to fully cool. Slice into four pieces and pour remaining melted butter over each.

**PER SERVING** Calories: 218

Protein: 7.2 G Fiber: 3.4 G Net Carbohydrates: 3.4G
Fat: 16.9 G

Sodium: 177 Mg Carbohydrates: 6.8 G Sugar: 2.1 G

# Radish Chips

Radishes might not come to mind right away when thinking about healthy, low-carb vegetables, but this recipe might just change that forever. This quick and healthy snack packs plenty of flavor as well as dietary fiber to help you feel full and avoid overeating.

- **Hands On Time**: 10 minutes

- **Cook Time**: 5 minutes

**Serves** 4

**Ingredients:**

- 2 cups water

- 1 pound radishes

- 1/4 teaspoon onion powder

- 1/4 teaspoon paprika

- 1/2 teaspoon garlic powder

- 2 tablespoons coconut oil, melted

## Directions

1. Place water in a medium saucepan and bring to a boil on stovetop.

2. Remove the top and bottom from each radish, then use a mandoline to slice each radish thin and uniformly. You may also use the slicing blade in the food processor for this step.

3. Place the radish slices into the boiling water for 5 minutes or until translucent.

4. Remove them from the water and place them into a clean kitchen towel to absorb excess moisture.

5. Toss the radish chips in a large bowl with remaining ingredients until fully coated in oil and seasoning.

6. Place radish chips into the air fryer basket.

7. Adjust the temperature to 320°F and set the timer for 5 minutes.

8. Shake the basket two or three times during the cooking time. Serve warm.

## PER SERVING

Calories: 77 Protein: 0.8 G Fiber: 1.8 G
Net Carbohydrates: 2.2 G Fat: 6.5 G Sodium: 40 Mg
Carbohydrates: 4.0 G Sugar: 2.0 G

# Flatbread

Flatbread is a great alternative for anything from a tortilla to a pizza crust. This easy recipe is flexible and versatile so you can make it any time of day to make your meal more filling.

- **Hands On Time**: 5 minutes

- **Cook Time**: 7 minutes

**Serves** 2

**Ingredients:**

- 1 cup shredded mozzarella cheese

- 4 cup blanched finely ground almond flour

- 1 ounce full-fat cream cheese, softened

### Directions

1. In a large microwave-safe bowl, melt mozzarella in the microwave for 30 seconds. Stir in almond flour until smooth and then add cream cheese. Continue mixing until dough forms, gently kneading it with wet hands if necessary.

2. Divide the dough into two pieces and roll out to V4" thickness between two pieces of parchment. Cut another piece of parchment to fit your air fryer basket.

3. Place a piece of flatbread onto your parchment and into the air fryer, working in two batches if needed.

4. Adjust the temperature to 320°F and set the timer for 7 minutes. Halfway through the cooking time flip the flatbread. Serve warm.

## PER SERVING

Calories: 296
Protein: 16.3 G Fiber: 1.5 G Net Carbohydrates: 3.3 G Fat: 22.6 G
Sodium: 402 Mg Carbohydrates: 4.8 G Sugar: 1.5 G

# Avocado Fries

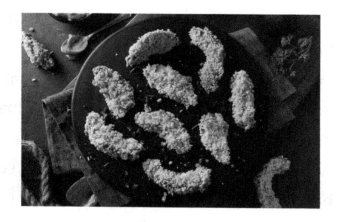

Avocados are an absolute staple on the keto diet. That's because they're low in carbs and very high in healthy fats that keep you full and focused. Some people like to eat avocados plain, but if you're not one of them, try these crispy Avocado Fries; they are a great, easy way to boost an avocado's flavor with little effort!

- **Hands On Time**: 15 minutes

- **Cook Time**: 5 minutes

**Serves** 4

## Ingredients:

- 2 medium avocados

- 1 ounce pork rinds, finely ground

### Directions

1. Cut each avocado in half. Remove the pit. Carefully remove the peel and then slice the flesh into 4"-thick slices.

2. Place the pork rinds into a medium bowl and press each piece of avocado into the pork rinds to coat completely. Place the avocado pieces into the air fryer basket.

3. Adjust the temperature to 350°F and set the timer for 5 minutes. Serve immediately.

## PER SERVING

Calories: 153
Protein: 5.4 G Fiber: 4.6 G
Net Carbohydrates: 1.3 G Fat: 11.9 G
Sodium: 121 Mg Carbohydrates: 5.9 G Sugar: 0.2 G

# Pita-Style Chips

You'll never miss the real thing with these chips! They come out amazingly crunchy and perfect for dipping! Try them with the Bacon Cheeseburger Dip (Chapter 3) or add some Mexican-style toppings for yummy nachos!

- **Hands On Time**: 10 minutes

- **Cook Time**: 5 minutes

**Serves** 4

- 1 cup shredded mozzarella cheese

- 1/2 ounce pork rinds, finely ground

- 1/4 cup blanched finely ground almond flour

- 1 large egg

  **Directions**

1. Place mozzarella in a large microwave-safe bowl and microwave for 30 seconds or until melted.
2. Add remaining ingredients and stir until a mostly smooth dough forms into a ball easily.

If dough is too hard, microwave for 15 seconds.

3. Roll dough out between two pieces of parchment into a large rectangle and then use a knife to cut triangle shaped chips. Place the chips into the air fryer basket.

4. Adjust the temperature to 350°F and set the timer for 5 minutes.

5. Chips will be golden in color and firm when done. As they cool, they will become even more firm.

**PER SERVING**

Calories: 161
Protein: 11.3 G Fiber: 0.8 G
Net Carbohydrates: 1.4 G Fat: 11.6 G
Sodium: 251 Mg Carbohydrates: 2.2 G Sugar: 0.6 G

# Roasted Eggplant

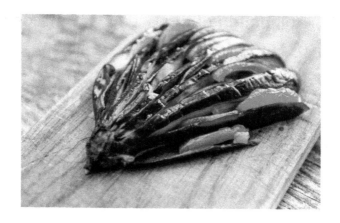

Eggplant is a very low-calorie vegetable that is high in fiber. This combination can be great for promoting weight loss, and luckily eggplant is very easy to add to your diet. This simple roasting method makes for a tasty side that would go great with other veggies or a yummy chicken dish.

- **Hands On Time**: 15 minutes

- **Cook Time**: 15 minutes

**Serves** 4

- 1 large eggplant

- 2 tablespoons olive oil

- 1/4 teaspoon salt

- 1/2 teaspoon garlic powder

## Directions

1. Remove top and bottom from eggplant. Slice eggplant into 1/4"-thick round slices.
2. Brush slices with olive oil. Sprinkle with salt and garlic powder. Place eggplant slices into the air fryer basket.
3. Adjust the temperature to 390°F and set the timer for 15 minutes.
4. Serve immediately.

## PER SERVING

Calories: 91
Protein: 1.3 G
Fiber: 3.7 G
Net Carbohydrates: 3.8 G Fat: 6.7 G Sodium: 147 Mg

Carbohydrates: 7.5 G Sugar: 4.4 G

# Parmesan Herb Focaccia Bread

This herb-baked focaccia substitute has only a fraction of carbs as the real thing, but it's the perfect sandwich bread to make sure you never feel left out while living your low-carb lifestyle.

- **Hands On Time**: 10 minutes

- **Cook Time**: 10 minutes

 **Serves** 6

**Ingredients:**

- 1 cup shredded mozzarella cheese

- 1 ounce full-fat cream cheese

- 1 cup blanched finely ground almond flour

- 1/4 cup ground golden flaxseed

- 1/4 cup grated Parmesan cheese

- 1/2 teaspoon baking soda

- 2 large eggs

- 1/2 teaspoon garlic powder

- 1/4 teaspoon dried basil

- 1/4 teaspoon dried rosemary

- 2 tablespoons salted butter, melted and divided

**Directions**

1. Place mozzarella, cream cheese, and almond flour into a large microwave-safe bowl and microwave for 1 minute. Add the flaxseed, Parmesan, and baking soda and stir until smooth ball forms. If the mixture cools too much, it will be hard to mix. Return to microwave for 10-15 seconds to rewarm if necessary.

2. Stir in eggs. You may need to use your hands to get them fully incorporated. Just keep stirring and they will absorb into the dough.

3. Sprinkle dough with garlic powder, basil, and rosemary and knead into dough. Grease a 6" round baking pan with 1 tablespoon melted butter. Press the dough evenly into the pan. Place pan into the air fryer basket.

4. Adjust the temperature to 400°F and set the timer for 10 minutes.

   At 7 minutes, cover with foil if bread begins to get too dark.

5. Remove and let cool at least 30 minutes. Drizzle with remaining butter and serve.

## PER SERVING

Calories: 292 Protein: 13.1 G Fiber: 4.0 G
Net Carbohydrates: 3.6 G Fat: 23.4 G Sodium: 370
Mg Carbohydrates: 7.6 G Sugar: 1.2 G

## SANDWICHES ARE BACK ON THE MENU!

For a filling meal, you can allow the bread to fully cool, then slice the entire round in half. Make it a club sandwich with turkey, bacon, lettuce, tomato, and mayo, or whatever your favorite toppings may be. Replace the top and slice into six pieces to serve. It's an easy meal for the whole family!

# Quick and Easy Home Fries

Jicama may seem like an intimidating vegetable from the outside but it's very easy to work with and well worth the extra effort. Peeling a jicama is a bit tricky but using a sharp knife to slice the peel off works easily. If you've never tasted it before, it's similar to a white potato in texture but with a hint of sweetness. It absorbs flavors easily, which makes jicama a good potato substitute. For a fraction of the carbs of the original, these home fries are the perfect smart swap for your keto diet.

• **Hands On Time**: 10 minutes

• **Cook Time**: 10 minutes

**Serves** 4

- 1 medium jicama, peeled

- 1 tablespoon coconut oil, melted

- 1/4 teaspoon ground black pepper

- 1/2 teaspoon pink Himalayan salt

- 1 medium green bell pepper, seeded and diced

- 1/2 medium white onion, peeled and diced

**Directions**

1. Cut jicama into 1" cubes. Place into a large bowl and toss with coconut oil until coated. Sprinkle with pepper and salt. Place into the air fryer basket with peppers and onion.
2. Adjust the temperature to 400°F and set the timer for 10 minutes.
3. Shake two or three times during cooking. Jicama will be tender and dark around edges. Serve immediately.

**PER SERVING**

Calories: 97 protein: 1.5 g fiber: 8.0 g
Net carbohydrates: 7.8 g fat: 3.3 g sodium: 202 mg
Carbohydrates: 15.8 g sugar: 4.0 g

# Jicama Fries

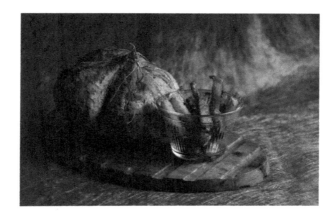

Jicama, also known as a Mexican potato, is a root vegetable native to Central and South America. A jicama is loaded with fiber, and it makes an excellent replacement for traditional French fries! One major selling point of air fryers is that they can get your French fries extremely crispy, with little to no oil. With this recipe you can take part in the fun, in a way that's much better for you!

- **Hands On Time**: 10 minutes

- **Cook Time**: 20 minutes

**Serves** 4

- 1 small jicama, peeled

- 3/4 teaspoon chili powder

- 1/4 teaspoon garlic powder

- 1/4 teaspoon onion powder

- 1/4 teaspoon ground black pepper

**Directions**

1. Cut jicama into matchstick-sized pieces.
2. Place pieces into a small bowl and sprinkle with remaining ingredients. Place the fries into the air fryer basket.
3. Adjust the temperature to 350°F and set the timer for 20 minutes. ✓ Toss the basket two or three times during cooking. Serve warm.

**PER SERVING**

Calories: 37

Protein: 0.8 G Fiber: 4.7 G

Net Carbohydrates: 4.0 G Fat: 0.1 G Sodium: 18 Mg

Carbohydrates: 8.7 G Sugar: 1.7 G

## WHERE CAN YOU FIND JICAMA?

Jicama is more common to grocery stores than you might realize! Check your produce aisle near regular potatoes, but if your search is unsuccessful be sure to try an international market.

# Fried Green Tomatoes

Green tomatoes are tomatoes that haven't fully ripened. Because of this, they're tarter than a red tomato and firmer. Fried Green Tomatoes are a sweet and juicy side that taste like summer with every bite and come together easily in your air fryer, so you don't have to worry about frying them in oil!

- **Hands On Time**: 10 minutes

- **Cook Time**: 7 minutes

**Serves** 4

- 2 medium green tomatoes

- 1 large egg

- 1/4 cup blanched finely ground almond flour

- 1/3 cup grated Parmesan cheese

**Directions**

1. Slice tomatoes into V2"-thick slices. In a medium bowl, whisk the egg. In a large

bowl, mix the almond flour and Parmesan.

2. Dip each tomato slice into the egg, then dredge in the almond flour mixture. Place the slices into the air fryer basket.

3. Adjust the temperature to 400°F and set the timer for 7 minutes.

4. Flip the slices halfway through the cooking time. Serve immediately.

## PER SERVING

Calories: 106

Protein: 6.2 g fiber: 1.4 g net carbohydrates: 4.5 g

fat: 6.7 g Sodium: 175 mg carbohydrates: 5.9 g

sugar: 2.8 g

# Fried Pickles

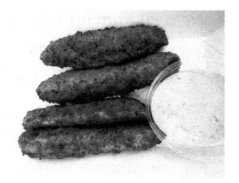

A favorite for many people in the Southern United States, Fried Pickles are a crispy and tart appetizer. They're traditionally battered with cornmeal and flour, but this keto-friendly alternative will give you all the flavor you need. Pair them with Southern "Fried" Chicken (Chapter 5) to keep the authentic Southern feel going!

- **Hands On Time**: 10 minutes

- **Cook Time**: 5 minutes

**Serves** 4

- 1 tablespoon coconut flour

- 1/3 cup blanched finely ground almond flour

- 1 teaspoon chili powder

- 1/4 teaspoon garlic powder

- 1 large egg

- 1 cup sliced pickles

## Directions

1. Whisk coconut flour, almond flour, chili powder, and garlic powder together in a medium bowl.
2. Whisk egg in a small bowl.
3. Pat each pickle with a paper towel and dip into the egg. Then dredge in the flour mixture. Place pickles into the air fryer basket.
4. Adjust the temperature to 400°F and set the timer for 5 minutes.
5. Flip the pickles halfway through the cooking time.

## PER SERVING

Calories: 85
Protein: 4.3 g fiber: 2.3 g
Net carbohydrates: 2.3 g fat: 6.1 g
Sodium: 351 mg carbohydrates: 4.6 g sugar: 1.2 g

# Potato Wedges

**Preparation time:** 10 minutes

**Cooking time:** 25 minutes

**Servings:** 4

**Ingredients:**

- 2 potatoes, cut into wedges
- 1 tablespoon olive oil
- Salt and black pepper to the taste
- 3 tablespoons sour cream
- 2 tablespoons sweet chili sauce

**Directions:**

1. In a bowl, mix potato wedges with oil, salt and pepper, toss well, add to air fryer's basket and cook at 360 degrees F for 25 minutes, flipping them once.
2. Divide potato wedges on plates, drizzle sour cream and chili sauce all over and serve them as a side dish. Enjoy!

**Nutrition:** calories 171, fat 8, fiber 9, carbs 18, protein 7

# Mushroom Side Dish

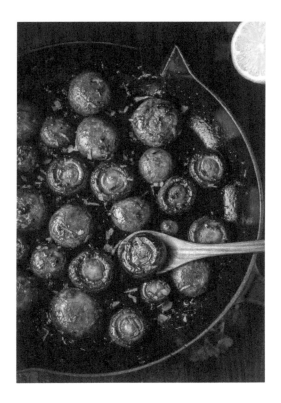

**Preparation time:** 10 minutes

**Cooking time:** 8 minutes

**Servings:** 4

**Ingredients:**

- 10 button mushrooms, stems removed 1 tablespoon Italian seasoning

- Salt and black pepper to the taste
- 2 tablespoons cheddar cheese, grated 1 tablespoon olive oil
- 2 tablespoons mozzarella, grated 1 tablespoon dill, chopped

## Directions:

1. In a bowl, mix mushrooms with Italian seasoning, salt, pepper, oil and dill and rub well.
2. Arrange mushrooms in your air fryer's basket, sprinkle mozzarella and cheddar in each and cook them at 360 degrees F for 8 minutes.
3. Divide them on plates and serve them as a side dish.

Enjoy!

**Nutrition:** calories 241, fat 7, fiber 8, carbs 14, protein 6

CPSIA information can be obtained
at www.ICGtesting.com
Printed in the USA
LVHW081550250421
685458LV00009B/483